Introduction

Welcome, intrepid seeker, to the threshold of a transformative odyssey—one that beckons you beyond the superficial promises of traditional fitness literature. This isn't just another guide; it's an invitation to embark on a profound journey toward holistic well-being, where health becomes not just a goal but an immersive way of life. Imagine a voyage that transcends the confines of conventional fitness routines, an exploration that touches the very core of your existence. As you turn the pages of this e-book, you're not merely delving into a manual; you're stepping into a realm where the principles of motivation and discipline intertwine to shape a narrative of lasting vitality and purpose.

In the luminous tapestry of this narrative, we're not fixated solely on the physical aspects of health. Instead, we're delving into the essence of motivation and discipline as catalysts for a broader transformation—one that encompasses your mental resilience, emotional balance, and spiritual fulfillment. Picture this journey as an intricate dance, where the rhythm of motivation propels you forward, and the structure of discipline provides the necessary framework for sustained progress. This isn't just about sculpting your body; it's about sculpting a life infused with meaning, passion, and a profound sense of well-being.

As you stand at the cusp of this exploration, envision the possibilities that lie ahead. This e-book isn't a prescription for a quick fix; it's a compass that points you toward a destination where every step is a conscious choice, and every choice contributes to the symphony of your holistic well-being. What awaits you within these pages is not a rigid set of rules but a flexible blueprint—one that adapts to your unique journey and celebrates the individuality of your pursuit.

Are you ready to redefine your narrative? To challenge the status quo of fitness literature and embrace a guide that transcends the mundane? The adventure unfolds with each word, each concept, and each revelation. This isn't just an e-book; it's an immersive experience—a journey where you are not a passive reader but an active participant, sculpting your destiny with every turn of the page.

So, fasten your seatbelt, dear reader, and prepare to dive into the depths of motivation and discipline, unlocking the doors to a life teeming with vitality, purpose, and the promise of an empowered transformation. The adventure begins now, and the possibilities are as boundless as your commitment to self-discovery and well-being. Welcome to a journey that goes beyond the ordinary, where health becomes a vibrant expression of your innermost aspirations. Let's embark on this odyssey together, weaving the tapestry of your extraordinary transformation—one chapter at a time.

Chapter 1: Understanding Motivation

Defining Motivation:

Welcome to the foundational chapter of your transformative journey, where we unravel the intricate layers of motivation—the pulsating life force that propels you forward. Beyond the conventional definitions, we plunge into the essence of motivation as a dynamic energy, a source of unwavering commitment that transcends mere desire. In this expansive exploration, we invite you to reflect on the dreams that resonate with the very core of your being, those aspirations that awaken a profound sense of purpose within you.

Motivation is more than a fleeting spark; it's a flame that burns brightly even in the face of adversity. As you delve into the multifaceted nature of motivation, consider it not as an external force but a reservoir of potential within you. It's the silent encouragement that whispers, "You can do it!" and the invisible hand that guides you through challenges. Through anecdotes, psychological insights, and real-life examples, we aim to redefine motivation as a deeply personal journey—one that transcends generic inspiration and taps into the unique wellspring of passion within each individual.

Different Types of Motivation:

Motivation wears a cloak of diversity, presenting itself in various forms to each individual. In this expansive section, we embark on a journey to distinguish between intrinsic and extrinsic motivation. Intrinsic motivation, stemming from your core values and genuine passion, becomes the heartbeat of your commitment. Extrinsic motivation, driven by external factors such as rewards or societal expectations, acts as a catalyst in the initial stages of your journey. Through engaging narratives and relatable scenarios, we guide you through the subtle dance between these motivations, emphasizing the significance of fostering a harmonious balance.

We delve into the psychology behind each type, understanding how the interplay between intrinsic and extrinsic motivations shapes your journey. By the end of this section, you'll not only identify the motivating forces within yourself but also appreciate how they can work synergistically to create a resilient, lasting commitment to your health and well-being.

The Psychology of Motivation:

Your mind is a powerful ally on this transformative journey, and understanding the psychology of motivation is akin to unlocking a treasure chest of self-awareness. Beyond theoretical concepts, we embark on a practical exploration of your mindset—how thoughts influence emotions, and emotions, in turn, guide actions. Through practical strategies and actionable insights, we empower you to cultivate a mindset that not only withstands challenges but also transforms them into stepping stones toward your goals.

This section delves into the role of self-talk, the impact of beliefs on motivation, and practical exercises to reframe negative thoughts. You'll gain a deeper understanding of the psychological mechanisms at play in your journey and emerge with a toolkit for cultivating a resilient and growth-oriented mindset. By the end of this chapter, you won't just understand motivation; you'll be equipped to harness its power effectively, setting the stage for a transformative journey toward a healthier and more vibrant you.

Chapter 2: Setting Goals

Importance of Setting Clear Goals:

In the vast expanse of your fitness journey, goals serve as the North Star, guiding you through the ebbs and flows of change. However, they are more than mere checkpoints; they are the crystallization of your aspirations, providing purpose and direction. This expansive section immerses you in the profound significance of setting clear and compelling goals. As you envision the life you desire, we guide you in distilling these visions into tangible, actionable goals. Each goal becomes a milestone, not just in your fitness journey but in the larger narrative of your life.

Through illustrative examples and practical exercises, we invite you to explore the depth of your aspirations. By clarifying your destination, you empower yourself to make intentional choices that align with your broader vision. Whether your goals involve weight loss, strength gain, or holistic well-being, this chapter is a roadmap for grounding your journey in clarity and purpose.

SMART Goal-Setting Principles:

Welcome to the transformative world of SMART goals—Specific, Measurable, Achievable, Relevant, and Time-bound. This section goes beyond conventional goal-setting, providing a deep dive into each principle to elevate your goal-setting game. Specific goals provide a clear trajectory, measurable goals offer tangible benchmarks, achievable goals fuel a sense of accomplishment, relevant goals align with your broader vision, and time-bound goals create a sense of urgency.

Through practical applications, real-life examples, and guided exercises, you'll not only grasp the theoretical framework of SMART goals but also learn how to infuse these principles into your personal journey. By the end of this section, your aspirations will transform from vague desires into actionable plans, setting the stage for a purposeful and intentional pursuit of a healthier and happier you.

Long-Term vs. Short-Term Goals:

In the grand tapestry of your fitness journey, long-term aspirations and short-term goals harmonize to create a symphony of progress. Long-term goals provide the overarching vision, the grand narrative that aligns with the life you envision. However, the beauty lies in the dance between the grand and the immediate—the long-term and the short-term. This section explores the delicate interplay between the two, emphasizing how short-term victories contribute to the grand melody of your overall well-being.

Through relatable anecdotes and practical strategies, we guide you in orchestrating a harmonious journey. Short-term goals become the vibrant strokes that infuse life into your daily routine, making the grand vision not just a distant dream but a tangible reality. By understanding and embracing the dynamic relationship between long-term aspirations and short-term goals, you'll cultivate a sustainable and fulfilling journey—one that unfolds in chapters of achievements and progress.

Chapter 3: Creating Objectives

Breaking Down Goals:

Your aspirations, while inspiring, may seem colossal at first glance. In this expansive exploration, we delve into the art of dissecting these ambitions into smaller, manageable objectives. Imagine these objectives as the foundation stones, forming a robust structure for your success. By breaking down your overarching goals into bite-sized, achievable tasks, you not only make progress more tangible but also unveil a roadmap that transforms ambitious visions into practical, actionable steps.

We guide you through the intricacies of identifying the key components of your goals, helping you articulate the specific actions required for success. This chapter encourages a shift from grandiose dreams to a systematic approach, laying the groundwork for sustained progress. With vivid examples and practical exercises, you'll gain proficiency in the art of breaking down goals, ensuring that every step is purposeful and propels you forward on your transformative journey.

The Significance of Small Wins:

In the intricate narrative of your fitness journey, small wins are not mere footnotes; they are the heartbeat of progress. This section is a deep dive into the profound impact of acknowledging and celebrating these victories. From completing a challenging workout to making a mindful dietary choice or maintaining consistency in your routine, each small win contributes to the narrative of success. Through relatable stories and motivational insights, we underscore the significance of recognizing these milestones as essential markers on your path.

By the end of this chapter, you'll develop a keen awareness of the power within small wins. They are not just moments of celebration but critical components of your journey, influencing your mindset and sustaining your motivation. This section is an ode to the journey, an invitation to revel in the joy of accomplishment, and a reminder that every step forward, no matter how small, is a testament to your commitment and dedication.

Tracking Progress and Celebrating Achievements:

Your journey is a living story, and every achievement is a chapter that deserves acknowledgment. In this expansive section, we delve into the art of tracking progress, offering insights into the importance of reflection and self-awareness. Learn practical strategies to monitor your advancements, whether through journaling, fitness apps, or other tracking methods. This chapter is not just about measuring physical changes; it's about cultivating a mindful approach that considers the holistic transformation—mind, body, and spirit.

Celebrating achievements takes center stage as we guide you through creating a personalized system of acknowledgment. By the end, you'll understand that tracking progress is not merely about numbers; it's a dynamic process that fosters self-discovery and reinforces your commitment. This chapter is a celebration of resilience, determination, and the evolving narrative of your transformation. It's an invitation to revel in your victories, both big and small, and recognize that each milestone is not just a destination but a checkpoint on your path to enduring well-being.

Chapter 4: Building Discipline

Understanding Discipline as a Key Factor:

Welcome to the core of your journey — the exploration of discipline as a key factor in achieving sustained success. Discipline is the backbone of your commitment, the unwavering force that propels you forward when motivation wavers. This extensive section delves into the multifaceted nature of discipline, emphasizing its role as the linchpin of a transformative lifestyle. By understanding discipline not as a rigid set of rules but as a flexible framework, you empower yourself to navigate challenges with resilience and grace.

We guide you through the nuances of discipline, illustrating its importance in maintaining consistency and fostering a positive mindset. Through real-life stories and practical strategies, you'll come to view discipline not as a restrictive force but as a liberating ally on your journey toward a healthier and more vibrant life.

Developing Habits for a Disciplined Lifestyle:

Discipline is not a fleeting commitment; it's a collection of habits that form the bedrock of your daily life. In this comprehensive exploration, we unravel the art of developing habits conducive to a disciplined lifestyle. Discover the science behind habit formation, the power of routines, and the role of positive reinforcement in cementing disciplined behaviors.

Through actionable tips and personalized exercises, you'll embark on a journey to cultivate habits that align with your goals. This chapter isn't about imposing rigid structures; it's about creating an environment that nurtures positive habits, making discipline an integral and sustainable part of your day-to-day existence.

Overcoming Common Obstacles to Discipline:

Discipline encounters roadblocks, but it's in overcoming these challenges that true strength emerges. This expansive section is a guide to identifying and surmounting common obstacles to discipline. Whether it's dealing with procrastination, managing time effectively, or navigating the pitfalls of perfectionism, we provide practical solutions to empower you on your journey.

By understanding that setbacks are not failures but opportunities for growth, you'll develop a resilient mindset that thrives in the face of challenges. This chapter serves as a compass, navigating you through the twists and turns of maintaining discipline, ensuring that even in moments of adversity, you stay firmly on the path to success.

Creating a Disciplined Mindset:

Discipline is not just external actions; it's a mindset that permeates every aspect of your being. In this profound exploration, we delve into the psychology of a disciplined mindset. Learn to cultivate self-control, resilience, and a positive outlook that fortifies your commitment. Through mindfulness practices and mindset-shifting exercises, you'll emerge with a disciplined mindset that extends beyond your fitness journey into all facets of your life.

This chapter is an invitation to view discipline as a dynamic and evolving aspect of your self-discovery. By embracing discipline as a mindset rather than a set of rules, you not only pave the way for success in your health and fitness journey but also lay the foundation for a disciplined and empowered life.

Chapter 5: Nurturing a Healthy Mindset

The Foundations of a Healthy Mindset:

Welcome to the heart of your holistic journey — the exploration of a healthy mindset as the cornerstone of enduring well-being. This profound chapter invites you to cultivate a mindset that not only sustains your health and fitness goals but also radiates positivity into every facet of your life. In understanding the foundations of a healthy mindset, we delve into the symbiotic relationship between thoughts, emotions, and actions.

This extensive section is not just about positive thinking; it's about fostering a mindset that thrives in resilience, embraces growth, and radiates self-compassion. Through practical exercises and insightful reflections, you'll embark on a transformative journey to redefine your relationship with yourself and the world around you.

Positive Self-Talk and Affirmations:

Your inner dialogue shapes your reality, and in this comprehensive exploration, we guide you through the art of positive self-talk and affirmations. Discover the power of language in influencing your mindset, and learn practical strategies to reframe negative thoughts into affirmations that bolster your self-esteem and motivation.

Through real-life examples and personalized exercises, you'll witness the transformative potential of cultivating a positive internal dialogue. This chapter is an invitation to become your own ally, speaking words of encouragement and empowerment that resonate with the journey you've embarked upon.

Embracing Resilience in the Face of Challenges:

A healthy mindset is not immune to challenges; instead, it thrives in resilience. This expansive section navigates the intricate terrain of embracing resilience as a fundamental aspect of your mental well-being. Explore the psychology of bouncing back from setbacks, developing coping strategies, and reframing obstacles as opportunities for growth.

Through engaging narratives and practical exercises, you'll cultivate a resilience that goes beyond your fitness journey, influencing how you navigate life's ups and downs. This chapter is a testament to the strength that emerges when a healthy mindset meets the inevitable challenges of the human experience.

Mindfulness and Present Living:

In the fast-paced rhythm of modern life, mindfulness becomes a beacon of serenity. This in-depth exploration introduces you to the transformative practice of mindfulness and present living. Learn to anchor yourself in the present moment, fostering a profound connection between mind and body.

Through mindfulness exercises and guided meditations, you'll cultivate a heightened awareness that extends into your health and fitness journey. This chapter is not just about stress reduction; it's an invitation to savor each moment, appreciating the richness of your journey and fostering a deep sense of fulfillment.

Cultivating Self-Compassion:

Amidst the pursuit of goals, it's crucial to cultivate self-compassion—a gentle and understanding approach to yourself. This extensive section delves into the art of self-compassion, exploring its transformative effects on your mindset and overall well-being. Learn to replace self-criticism with kindness, acknowledging that imperfections are an integral part of the human experience.

Through self-compassion exercises and reflective practices, you'll develop a nurturing relationship with yourself. This chapter is an invitation to be your own supporter, recognizing that the journey is as much about self-discovery and growth as it is about achieving specific goals.

Chapter 6: The Transformative Power of Nutrition

Unveiling the Essence of Nutrition:

Welcome to the realm where nourishment becomes the catalyst for your transformation. This chapter delves into the transformative power of nutrition, recognizing it not just as a means to an end but as a cornerstone of your holistic well-being. We embark on a journey to unveil the essence of nutrition — a journey that transcends dieting trends and embraces the profound impact of food on your body, mind, and spirit.

In this extensive exploration, we unravel the science behind nutrition, demystifying the roles of macronutrients, micronutrients, and their intricate interplay within your body. Beyond the caloric lens, we invite you to see food as a source of vitality, a nourishing elixir that fuels your journey toward optimal health.

Crafting a Balanced and Sustainable Diet:

Nutrition isn't about restriction; it's about crafting a balanced and sustainable diet that aligns with your health and fitness goals. This comprehensive section guides you through the art of creating a diet that not only meets your nutritional needs but also complements your lifestyle. We explore the principles of balance, variety, and moderation, ensuring that your relationship with food is not just nourishing but also enjoyable.

Through practical tips, meal planning strategies, and delicious recipes, you'll discover the joy of savoring nutrient-dense foods. This chapter is an invitation to foster a positive relationship with nutrition, making informed choices that contribute to your overall well-being.

Understanding the Psychological Aspects of Eating:

Beyond the biochemical aspects, eating is a psychological experience intimately connected to emotions, habits, and cultural influences. This in-depth exploration sheds light on the psychological aspects of eating, guiding you to develop a mindful and intuitive relationship with food. Explore the impact of emotional eating, uncover strategies to break free from unhealthy patterns, and learn to savor the sensory pleasures of eating.

Through mindfulness exercises and reflective practices, you'll cultivate awareness around your eating habits. This chapter is not just about what you eat but also how you eat—a holistic approach that considers the mental and emotional dimensions of nourishment.

Tailoring Nutrition to Your Unique Needs:

Your body is unique, and so are its nutritional needs. This extensive section is a guide to tailoring nutrition to your individual requirements, taking into account factors such as age, gender, activity level, and specific health goals. Discover personalized approaches to dietary patterns, whether you're aiming for weight management, muscle gain, or overall well-being.

Through practical assessments and expert insights, you'll gain a deeper understanding of how to customize your nutrition plan. This chapter is an invitation to embrace your individuality, recognizing that there's no one-size-fits-all approach to nourishment.

Embracing a Lifelong Approach to Nutrition:

Nutrition is not a short-term fix; it's a lifelong commitment to your health and well-being. This final section of the chapter is a journey into embracing a lifelong approach to nutrition. We explore the concept of food as a source of pleasure, connection, and cultural richness. Learn to navigate social situations, celebrate special occasions, and indulge in occasional treats while maintaining a balanced and sustainable relationship with food.

Through actionable tips and real-life examples, you'll emerge with the tools to navigate the complexities of the modern food landscape. This chapter is a celebration of the joy of eating, a recognition that a lifelong commitment to nutrition is not a rigid constraint but a liberating choice that enhances the quality of your life.

Chapter 7: The Holistic Approach to Exercise

Rediscovering the Joy of Movement:

Welcome to a chapter that redefines exercise not as a chore but as a celebration of the joy of movement. In this expansive exploration, we delve into the holistic approach to exercise, transcending the confines of traditional fitness routines. Rediscover the pleasure inherent in physical activity as we guide you through the transformative power of movement for your body, mind, and spirit.

In the journey to rediscover the joy of movement, we unravel the science behind exercise, exploring its profound impact on cardiovascular health, muscular strength, and mental well-being. This chapter is an invitation to shift your perspective from viewing exercise as a task to embracing it as a dynamic and pleasurable expression of vitality.

Crafting a Personalized Fitness Plan:

Exercise is not a one-size-fits-all endeavor; it's a personalized journey tailored to your unique needs and goals. This comprehensive section is a guide to crafting a personalized fitness plan that aligns with your aspirations. We explore the principles of cardiovascular exercise, strength training, flexibility, and the importance of incorporating variety into your routine.

Through personalized assessments and expert insights, you'll gain clarity on the type of exercise that suits your body and lifestyle. This chapter is an invitation to embrace the diversity of movement, recognizing that your fitness plan should be an enjoyable and sustainable expression of self-care.

Exploring Mind-Body Practices:

Beyond traditional forms of exercise, this in-depth exploration introduces you to mind-body practices that bridge the gap between physical and mental well-being. Dive into the transformative realms of yoga, tai chi, and mindfulness-based exercises. These practices not only enhance your physical fitness but also foster mental clarity, emotional balance, and a profound sense of connection.

Through guided practices and experiential insights, you'll discover the holistic benefits of integrating mind-body exercises into your routine. This chapter is an invitation to explore the synergy between body and mind, recognizing that true well-being encompasses both physical and mental vitality.

Navigating Challenges and Building Consistency:

Embarking on a fitness journey inevitably encounters challenges, and building consistency is a key to success. This expansive section is a guide to navigating challenges and establishing habits that stand the test of time. Explore strategies to overcome common obstacles, develop resilience in the face of setbacks, and build a consistent exercise routine that becomes an integral part of your lifestyle.

Through real-life stories and practical tips, you'll gain insights into creating a sustainable relationship with exercise. This chapter is an invitation to view challenges not as roadblocks but as stepping stones, recognizing that building consistency is a journey of self-discovery and growth.

Fostering a Positive Relationship with Exercise:

Exercise is not solely about physical transformation; it's an opportunity to foster a positive and empowering relationship with your body. This final section of the chapter is a journey into nurturing a positive mindset around exercise. We explore the concept of joyful movement, Intuitive exercise, and embracing your body's capabilities without judgment.

Through self-reflection exercises and motivational insights, you'll emerge with a renewed perspective on exercise—one that celebrates your body, acknowledges your progress, and cultivates a sense of gratitude for the transformative power of movement. This chapter is a celebration of the profound connection between your body, mind, and the joy that arises when you move with purpose and self-compassion.

Chapter 8: The Importance of Rest and Recovery

Redefining Rest as a Vital Component:

Welcome to a chapter that redefines rest from a mere pause between activities to a vital component of your holistic well-being. In this extensive exploration, we delve into the importance of rest and recovery as essential pillars of a sustainable and thriving lifestyle. Rediscover the art of slowing down and rejuvenating, recognizing that rest is not a sign of weakness but a strategic investment in your physical, mental, and emotional resilience.

As we unravel the science behind rest, you'll gain insights into the physiological and psychological benefits that come from adequate recovery. This chapter is an invitation to shift your mindset, viewing rest not as a passive state but as an active and intentional practice that enhances your overall health.

Understanding the Science of Sleep:

Sleep is a cornerstone of optimal well-being, yet its significance is often overlooked. This comprehensive section is a guide to understanding the science of sleep and its profound impact on your physical and mental health. Explore the different stages of sleep, the role of circadian rhythms, and practical strategies to enhance the quality of your sleep.

Through evidence-based insights and actionable tips, you'll develop a deeper appreciation for the transformative power of a good night's sleep. This chapter is an invitation to prioritize and cultivate healthy sleep habits, recognizing that adequate rest is the foundation upon which your health and vitality thrive.

Incorporating Active Recovery:

Recovery is not synonymous with inactivity; it's an active and intentional process. This in-depth exploration introduces you to the concept of active recovery — a dynamic approach that promotes healing and rejuvenation through purposeful movement. We explore the benefits of activities like yoga, gentle stretching, and low-intensity exercises in enhancing recovery.

Through practical exercises and expert guidance, you'll discover how active recovery complements your fitness routine, prevents burnout, and accelerates the restoration of your body. This chapter is an invitation to embrace the synergy between movement and recovery, recognizing that a balanced approach is key to sustained well-being.

Managing Stress and Building Resilience:

In the modern pace of life, stress has become ubiquitous, affecting both physical and mental health. This expansive section is a guide to managing stress and building resilience through intentional rest practices. Explore mindfulness, meditation, and stress-reducing techniques that empower you to navigate life's challenges with grace and poise.

Through experiential practices and expert insights, you'll cultivate resilience — the ability to bounce back from stress and adversity. This chapter is an invitation to view stress not as an insurmountable obstacle but as an opportunity for growth and self-discovery.

Balancing Work and Rest:

Finding the delicate balance between work and rest is an art that contributes to overall well-being. This final section of the chapter is a journey into creating a harmonious relationship between your active pursuits and restful moments. Explore practical strategies for time management, setting boundaries, and fostering a lifestyle that honors the ebb and flow of energy.

Through real-life examples and reflective exercises, you'll emerge with a personalized approach to balancing work and rest. This chapter is an invitation to cultivate a lifestyle that honors both productivity and rejuvenation, recognizing that a well-rested individual is a resilient and empowered individual.

Conclusion:

Embracing the Journey Towards Holistic Well-Being

Congratulations on reaching the culmination of this transformative journey towards holistic well-being! This concluding chapter is not just an endpoint but a stepping stone to a life enriched with vitality, purpose, and enduring health. As we reflect on the chapters that unfolded, it's essential to recognize that true well-being extends beyond physical fitness; it encompasses the intricate interplay of mind, body, and spirit.

In this extensive exploration, you've ventured into the realms of motivation and discipline, discovering the dynamic forces that propel you toward lasting change. You've embraced the art of setting goals and creating objectives, crafting a roadmap that aligns with your deepest aspirations. The psychology of motivation and the significance of a disciplined mindset have been unveiled, providing you with the tools to navigate challenges and celebrate victories.

Your journey continued with a holistic approach to nutrition, where food became a source of nourishment, pleasure, and cultural richness. Crafting a balanced and sustainable diet became not just a choice but a celebration of your unique body and its needs. The transformative power of nutrition emerged as a key element in sculpting a life infused with energy and well-being.

The exploration of exercise went beyond conventional fitness routines, inviting you to rediscover the joy of movement. Crafting a personalized fitness plan tailored to your individual needs became a testament to the diversity of physical activity and its potential for holistic growth. Mind-body practices illuminated the interconnectedness of physical and mental well-being, introducing a harmonious blend of movement and mindfulness into your daily routine.

The importance of rest and recovery unfolded as essential components of a thriving lifestyle. You learned to view rest not as a passive state but as an intentional practice that enhances your resilience and overall health. The science of sleep, the dynamic approach of active recovery, and stress management techniques equipped you with the knowledge and tools to navigate the intricate dance between activity and rejuvenation.

As you stand at this crossroads of completion, it's vital to recognize that well-being is not a destination but a continual journey. The chapters you've explored serve as a foundation, providing you with insights, strategies, and practices to navigate the path ahead. Your commitment to holistic well-being is a lifelong endeavor, a commitment to nurturing the symbiotic relationship between your mind, body, and spirit.

Next Steps:

Crafting Your Continued Journey

The conclusion of this e-book marks the beginning of your continued journey towards holistic well-being. Here are personalized next steps to guide you in crafting a path that aligns with your goals and aspirations:

Reflect on Your Journey: Take a moment to reflect on the insights and practices that resonated most with you. Consider how these learnings can be integrated into your daily life to foster lasting change.

Set Evolving Goals: Goals are not static; they evolve with your journey. Reassess your aspirations, refine your objectives, and set new goals that align with your current phase of growth.

Create Your Holistic Blueprint: Craft a holistic blueprint that incorporates the principles of motivation, discipline, nutrition, exercise, and rest into your lifestyle. This personalized plan will serve as a compass, guiding your choices and actions.

Cultivate Mindfulness: Integrate mindfulness into your daily routine. Whether through meditation, mindful eating, or conscious movement, mindfulness enhances your awareness and connection with the present moment.

Prioritize Self-Care: Recognize that self-care is not a luxury but a necessity. Prioritize rest, recovery, and activities that bring you joy. The more you nurture yourself, the more resilient you become in facing life's challenges.

Celebrate Progress: Acknowledge and celebrate your progress, no matter how small. Each step forward is a testament to your commitment to holistic well-being. Use milestones as opportunities for reflection and celebration.

Seek Support: Embark on this journey with a sense of community and support. Share your goals with friends, family, or a mentor who can provide encouragement, accountability, and companionship along the way.

Embrace Adaptability: Life is dynamic, and your well-being journey should be adaptable. Embrace change, be open to trying new approaches, and cultivate a mindset that views challenges as opportunities for growth.

Remember, this is your unique journey, and you have the power to shape it according to your aspirations. The chapters explored in this e-book are foundational, but the story of your well-being is an evolving narrative—one that unfolds with each intentional choice, each moment of mindfulness, and each step towards lasting health and vitality.

As you step into the next chapter of your journey, may it be filled with a sense of purpose, resilience, and the unwavering belief that holistic well-being is not just a destination but a way of life. Here's to your continued growth, vitality, and the extraordinary story you are crafting—one chapter at a time.